Routledge Revivals

CONSTITUTION AND HEALTH

CONSTITUTION AND HEALTH

BY

RAYMOND PEARL

**Professor of Biology
in The Johns Hopkins University, Baltimore**

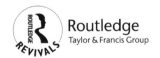

Routledge
Taylor & Francis Group

First published in 1933 by Kegan Paul, Trench, Trubner & Co., Ltd

This edition first published in 2018 by Routledge
2 Park Square, Milton Park, Abingdon, Oxon, OX14 4RN

and by Routledge
711 Third Avenue, New York, NY 10017

Routledge is an imprint of the Taylor & Francis Group, an informa business

© 1933 Taylor & Francis

Publisher's Note
The publisher has gone to great lengths to ensure the quality of this reprint but points out that some imperfections in the original copies may be apparent.

Disclaimer
The publisher has made every effort to trace copyright holders and welcomes correspondence from those they have been unable to contact.
A Library of Congress record exists under ISBN: 34030904

ISBN 13: 978-1-138-55493-1 (hbk)
ISBN 13: 978-1-315-12293-9 (ebk)

PSYCHE MINIATURES
General Series No. 60

CONSTITUTION AND HEALTH

PSYCHE MINIATURES
2/6 Net

MEDICAL

Migraine	F. G. Crookshank, M.D., F.R.C.P.
Aphasia	S. A. Kinnier Wilson, M.D., F.R.C.P.
Rheumatic Diseases	M. B. Ray, D.S.O., M.D.
Types of Mind and Body	E. Miller, M.B., M.R.C.S., D.P.M.
Dermatological Neuroses	W. J. O'Donovan, O.B.E., M.D.
Diagnosis: and Spiritual Healing	F. G. Crookshank, M.D.
Medicine: and the Man	Millais Culpin, M.D., F.R.C.S.
Idiosyncrasies	Sir Humphry Rolleston, *Bart.*, G.C.V.O., K.C.B.
The Constitutional Factor	Arthur F. Hurst, M.D., F.R.C.P.
The Troubled Conscience	Professor C. Blondel
Mirror-Writing	Macdonald Critchley, M.D., F.R.C.P.
Hypochondria	R. D. Gillespie, M.D., M.R.C.P., D.P.M
Individual Diagnosis	F. G. Crookshank, M.D., F.R.C.P
Individual Sexual Problems	F. G. Crookshank, M.D., F.R.C.P.

GENERAL

Science and Poetry	I. A. Richards
Over-Population	P. Sargant Florence
Man Not A Machine	Eugenio Rignano
The Hunter in Our Midst	R. Lowe Thompson
Fee, Fi, Fo, Fum	H. J. Massingham
Myth in Primitive Psychology	B. Malinowski
The Father in Primitive Psychology	B. Malinowski
On History	A. L. Rowse
Economics and Human Behaviour	P. Sargant Florence
Fatalism or Freedom	C. Judson Herrick
Emergent Evolution	W. Morton Wheeler
Man A Machine	Joseph Needham
Intelligence	Claude A. Claremont
The Basis of Memory	W. R. Bousfield
Selene, or Sex and the Moon	H. Munro Fox
The Standardization of Error	Vilhjalmur Stefansson
The Alchemy of Light and Colour	Oliver L. Reiser
Culture: A Symposium	Elliot Smith and others
The Battle of Behaviorism	Watson and McDougall
Outline of Comparative Psychology	C. J. Warden
The Notation of Movement	Margaret Morris
Mescal	H. Klüver
Prodigal Sons	Montgomery Evans
The Future of the Earth	Harold Jeffreys
Uplift in Economics	P. Sargant Florence
The Conquest of Thought by Invention	H. S. Hatfield
A Philosophy in Outline	E. S. Bennett
Ghosts and Spirits in the Ancient World	E. J. Dingwall
The Structure of Insanity	Trigant Burrow
Phyloanalysis	William Galt
Interpretation and Analysis	J. Wisdom
International Communication	Shenton and others
Opposition	C. K. Ogden
Jeremy Bentham, 1832—2032	C. K. Ogden
Word Economy	L. W. Lockhart
Symbolic Distance	S. Buchanan
Carl and Anna (in Basic English)	Leonhard Frank
International Talks (in Basic English)	Wickham Steed
*Basic English**	C. K. Ogden

* For other books on Basic English, see end page.

PUBLISHED IN CONNECTION WITH
PSYCHE
An Annual Review of General and Applied Psychology

CONSTITUTION AND HEALTH

BY

RAYMOND PEARL

Professor of Biology
in The Johns Hopkins University, Baltimore

LONDON:
KEGAN PAUL, TRENCH, TRUBNER & Co. Ltd.
BROADWAY HOUSE, CARTER LANE E.C.
1933

OTHER BOOKS BY RAYMOND PEARL

Modes of Research in Genetics.

Diseases of Poultry. Their Etiology, Diagnosis, Treatment and Prevention. (With F. M. Surface and M. R. Curtis).

The Nation's Food. A Statistical Study of a Physiological and Social Problem. (Out of Print).

The Biology of Death. (Swedish Translation: *Liv Och Dod*).

Introduction to Medical Biometry and Statistics. (Revised Edition, 1930).

Studies in Human Biology.

The Biology of Population Growth.

Alcohol and Longevity. (German translation: *Alkohol und Lebensdauer*).

To Begin With. (Revised Edition, 1930).

The Present Status of Eugenics.

The Rate of Living.

Printed in Great Britain by
R. I. SEVERS, CAMBRIDGE

CONTENTS

		PAGE
I.	DISEASE	9
II.	CLASSIFICATIONS	17
III.	CONSTITUTION	33
IV.	SOMATOLOGY	51
V.	HEALTH	68
VI.	CONCLUSION	83
VII.	NOTES AND REFERENCES	90

ILLUSTRATIONS

TEXT FIGURES

FIG.   PAGE

1. Trends of mortality with age,
   according to organ systems (A)
   in direct contact with environment, and (B) not in direct
   contact   31

2. Chart of factors concerned in
   constitution   46

3. Diagram to illustrate the biological   57
   conception of bodily habitus   .

4. Scales used in grading somato-
   logical types   65

PLATES

PLATE   FACING PAGE

I.   Rear View of two women.   A.
     Asthenic. B. Pyknic   .   .   53

II. Individual B of Plate I enlarged to
     the same total height as A   .   59

III. Individual B of Plate I enlarged to
     have the same leg length as A .   60

IV. Individual B of Plate I reduced to
     have the same chest breadth as A   61

V.   Rear view of two dysplastic
     women   64

PREFACE

The material in this book is an expansion of a lecture given at the Army Medical Center, Washington, D.C., on May 15, 1933. I have thought it best to leave it in the somewhat informal discourse of the lecture platform. References to the literature, and other annotations, are numbered consecutively and placed together at the end of the book.

It should be pointed out here at the start, as it is in the text, that the author is not a medical man, but merely a biologist greatly interested in human biology; aware of his deficiencies in knowledge and experience consequent upon not having pursued a medical career; but with an equally lively sense of his inalienable right as a biologist to study man, the most interesting of all animals.

RAYMOND PEARL.

Baltimore, July, 1933.

I

DISEASE

The idea that a man's biological constitution—his morphological structure, his physiological functioning, and his mental and emotional make-up—has something to do with his state of health in general and his illnesses in particular is as old as medicine itself. Indeed some of the earliest writers on such matters, whose works may be regarded as still maintaining in some degree an unbroken continuity with the present-day body of medical doctrine, appear to have had a clearer insight than characterizes a not inconsiderable part of the thinking of physicians to-day as to the importance of the innate constitution of the individual as a causal factor in determining his state of health. The *Airs, Waters, and Places* of Hippocrates as an example is, above everything else, a biological discussion of the inseparable effects of nature and nurture (constitution and environment) in making individuals

and races what they are observed to be.[1]
In illustration the following passage may
be quoted (Chaps. 20 and 21) : [2]

" I will give you a strong proof of the humidity
[laxity] of their constitutions. You will find the
greater part of the Scythians, and all the
Nomades, with marks of the cautery on their
shoulders, arms, wrists, breasts, hip-joints, and
loins, and that for no other reason but the
humidity and flabbiness of their constitution,
for they can neither strain with their bows, nor
launch the javelin from their shoulders owing
to their humidity and atony ; but when they are
burnt, much of the humidity in their joints is
dried up, and they become better braced, better
fed, and their joints get into a more suitable
condition. They are flabby and squat at first,
because, as in Egypt, they are not swathed ;
and then they pay no attention to horsemanship,
so that they may be adepts at it ; and because of
their sedentary mode of life ; for the males, when
they cannot be carried about on horseback, sit
the most of their time in the wagon, and rarely
practise walking, because of their frequent
migrations and shiftings of situation ; and as to
the women, it is amazing how flabby and
sluggish they are. The Scythian race are tawny
from the cold, and not from the intense heat of
the sun, for the whiteness of the skin is parched
by the cold, and becomes tawny.

It is impossible that persons of such a
constitution could be prolific, for, with the man,
the sexual desires are not strong, owing to the
laxity of his constitution, the softness and
coldness of his belly, from all which causes it is
little likely that a man should be given to venery ;
and besides, from being jaded by exercise on
horseback, the men become weak in their desires.
On the part of the men these are the causes ;
but on that of the women, they are embonpoint
and humidity ; for the womb cannot take in the
semen, nor is the menstrual discharge such as

10

it should be, but scanty and at too long intervals; and the mouth of the womb is shut up by fat and does not admit the semen; and, moreover, they themselves are indolent and fat, and their bellies cold and soft. From these causes the Scythian race is not prolific. Their female servants furnish a strong proof of this; for they no sooner have connection with a man than they prove with child, owing to their active course of life and the slenderness of body ".

It is not a matter of great importance as to whether the Hippocratic treatise is meticulously ' right ' or not in respect of the observations upon which the discussion just quoted (or other similar ones that might have been used as an example) is based. The important things are the perception of the problem involved, and the manner of approach to its solution. We see clearly the sure insight which philosophically grounds an immediately medical discussion upon a broad, general biological base.

It is not, however, my purpose on this occasion to trace the history of ideas on the subject of constitution, intrinsically interesting as that history is. What I wish rather to do is to discuss the ancient problem of the relation of human constitution to disease from the point of view of modern biology. Not being a medical man I can only speak of these matters in the same sort of way that a biologist deals with his problems in organisms lower in the evolutionary scale than man. While this restriction perhaps makes for a certain detachment, possibly having its valuable points, it also sets definite limits about the universe of discourse. It furthermore emphasizes, and indeed in a sense necessitates somewhat contrasting points of view.

The biologist who interests himself at all in the subject of pathology looks primarily upon disease merely as one part of the general biology of the organism. He thinks of it first as an interesting aberration from the usual normal and integrated functioning of the whole organism, rather than as a specific, discrete, inimical entity, fastening on its victim as it were. One gathers that medical men in the practical conduct of their business commonly tend, perhaps only for convenience, to think of a disease, say pneumonia, as ' attacking ' a man. The physician's function is often described as that of ' combatting ' it, or, if possible of ' preventing ' it. We read and hear of ' invaders ', and sometimes the nature of such expressions is such as to carry something of the implication that the ' invaders ' are acting with a purpose, that purpose being the laying low of the unfortunate victim. It is not intended to imply that intelligent and thoughtful physicians seriously regard such views as giving a complete picture of the nature of disease. But that such teleological ideas do, consciously or subconsciously, play a considerable rôle in everyday practical medical thinking is, in fact, undeniable.[3]

The biologist's way of looking at the matter is in sharp contrast to this, possibly in part because he does not come into first-hand contact with the details of the business except when he, himself in person, is ' invaded '. In general, and when personally feeling well, he tends to think of a disease, say again pneumonia, as a curious and profound alteration in the usual normal functioning of the human organism associated with a disturbance in a normally equilibrated and therefore unnoticed commensalism between man and a particular lower plant. For him, in short, the alteration of the biology of the organism (man) *is* the disease. This idea would seem to have occurred to Galen, although some, at least, of his followers developed a somewhat different philosophy of the matter. In the *Natural Faculties*[4]

(II, ix) he says : " Are you, then, going to oppose those who maintain that the function of every organ is a natural eucrasia, that the dyscrasia is itself known as a *disease*, and that it is certainly by this that the activity becomes impaired? "

It is of interest to note in passing that Aristotle had expressed the biological essence of Galen's eucrasia, as the following passage shows : [5]

" And the animal organism must be conceived after the similitude of a well-governed common-wealth. When order is once established in it there is no more need of a separate monarch to preside over each several task. The individuals each play their assigned part as it is ordered, and one thing follows another in its accustomed order. So in animals there is the same orderliness —nature taking the place of custom—and each part naturally doing its own work as nature has composed them. There is no need then of a soul in each part, but she resides in a kind of central governing place of the body, and the remaining parts live by continuity of natural structure, and play the parts Nature would have them play ".

The discovery of all or even the more important of the underlying causes for the functional alteration or dyscrasia which is disease constitutes a major biological problem. The biologist would approach this problem with an entirely open mind as to the relative importance of endogenous (innate, constitutional) and exogenous (external, environmental) factors in the

14

case, as Hippocrates did. But his whole previous experience with problems similar in their nature would lead him confidently to expect that in the end both sets of factors would be found to be involved. He would further expect, of course, that in some diseases the exogenous factors might be more important than the endogenous, while in other diseases the reverse might be the case, but it would certainly never occur to him to expect that in any disease the influence of one of these sets of factors would be *wholly* wanting. In his experience living nature does not act that way about anything.

I suppose that most enlightened physicians of the present day would say, if asked, that this expresses exactly their own view. And so it undoubtedly does, provided the discourse is kept with scrupulous care upon that high plane of platitudinous generality which enables statesmen to exude wisdom as a tapped tree does sap. The difficulties and differences appear when we come down to particular cases. Lip service to a general idea is one thing ; the carrying over of the logically necessary implications and consequences of that general idea to a particular case where it encounters firmly entrenched and vested intellectual interests in possession of the property, as it were, is quite another and less easy matter. When one of the foremost clinicians in the world to-day, a man of deep learning and broad experience, can say :[6] " En sorte qu'au total, nous sommes menés à la conclusion que les faits, aussi bien les faits anciens que les faits nouveaux, ne permettent pas de considérer l'hérédité comme un facteur de propagation de la tuberculose ", it seems to me that there *is* in fact a gap between the thinking of current medicine and current biology that has not yet been fully bridged.

II

CLASSIFICATIONS

The biological view of the matter leads to the simplest and most general of possible theoretical classifications of disease, as follows :

Any disease or pathological process is, in its origin or causation, either

1. Chiefly exogenous — Primarily due to (A) infections, infestations or traumatisms, with the constitution of the individual playing a relatively unimportant rôle.

2. Chiefly endogenous — Primarily due to (B) general or specific constitutional peculiarities, with infections, etc. playing a relatively unimportant rôle.

3. Both exogenous and endogenous — Due to mutual interactions of (A) and (B), both playing important, though not necessarily equal, rôles.

This classification tends to throw into strong relief the difference in the outlook of the medical man and the biologist upon disease. The medical man tends to think of particular diseases as falling for the most part definitely into Class 1 of this

17

scheme, with a very small minority sometimes somewhat reluctantly admitted, on the basis of presently inadequate knowledge, to fall definitely into Class 2 ; the biologist inclines rather to think that, if more were known about the matter than in fact is, what are called particular specific diseases would mostly be found to belong to Class 3.

But this is an extremely general classification, and because of its generality of no great significance. Considered as a scientific method, however, classification is of prime importance. It has been rightly called the most fundamental, as well as the first, of all scientific methods. There have been many and various classifications of diseases in the history of medicine, and there will doubtless be many more. Nosology does not now enjoy the vogue that it has in times past, but it is a subject that never dies.

While some of the special classifications of disease have been completely logical, others, like the International List of the Causes of Death used in tabulation of mortality returns by vital statisticians, are naively and grossly illogical, in that they shift *in medias res* from one basis of classification, say etiological, to another, say organological. This classification includes, for example, as major headings, such logically disparate sub-universes as (*a*) Infectious and Parasitic Diseases, and (*b*) Diseases of the Respiratory System. Here obviously some *a*'s are *b*, and some *b*'s are *a*. But in a completely logical classification no *a* can be *b*, and no *b* can be *a*.

In the history of medicine logical classifications of disease have been variously and sometimes curiously based. Perhaps what is likely to be regarded by medical men as a superlatively odd classification is the one made by the great Linnaeus, the founder of plant and animal taxonomy. It tends to be forgotten that he was professionally a medical man, and that he classified diseases, as well as the organisms that suffered from them. But he did. His *Genera Morborum*[7] (1759) grouped all diseases into eleven classes, *upon the basis of the symptoms they exhibited*.

The classes were as follows :

MORBI

			Exanthematici.	I.
Febriles (e sanguine in medullam)...			Critici.	II.
			Phlogistici.	III.
		Sensationis	Dolorosi.	IV.
	Nervii	Judicii	Mentales.	V.
		Motus	Quietales.	VI.
			Motorii.	VII.
Morbi	Fluidi Secretionis.		Suppressorii.	VIII.
(Temperati)			Evacuatorii.	IX.
	Solidi	Interni	Deformes.	X.
		Externi	Vitia.	XI.

EXANTHEMATICI. Febris cum efflorescentia cutis maculata.
CRITICI. Febris cum urinae hypostasi lateritia.
PHLOGISTICI. Febris cum pulsu duro, dolore topico.
DOLOROSI. Doloris sensatio.
MENTALES. Judicii alienatio.
QUIETALES. Motus abolitio.
MOTORII. Motus involuntarius.
SUPPRESSORII. Meatum impeditio.
EVACUATORII. Fluidorum evacuatio.
DEFORMES. Solidorum facies mutata.
VITIA. Externa palpabilia.

Egdahl[7] suggests that the last two classes represent a shift from the symptomological base to a morphological, and implies that in so far Linnaeus slipped in his usually sure-footed logic. But this was certainly not the view of Linnaeus himself. The deformities on the one hand and the externally palpable tumors, fractures, etc. on the other, were for him *symptoms* of particular pathological conditions, just as much as exanthematous fevers were. The most interesting thing about this classification is not its oddity to present-day medical modes of thinking, but the fact that its philosophical foundation is strictly biological. If disease is an alteration (dyscrasia) of the normally integrated and smoothly running organic system, what could be more logical than to classify diseases upon the basis of the observable manifestations of the alterations, which is exactly what symptoms are ? The usefulness of the classification is, of course, another and quite different matter. Its philosophy, however, cannot be impugned.

But all this is a digression. My primary purpose in discussing the classification of diseases is to direct attention to a particular biological classification of diseases, designed specifically for the purpose of aiding in a logical approach to the problems of constitution. It is based upon the principle of assigning each disease (or, actually, " cause of death " as recognized in the International List), in so far as present knowledge on the one hand and official modes of tabulation on the other make it possible, to that organ system of the body whose failure to function normally (dyscrasia) leads to death.[8] The underlying idea of this arrangement is to put all those lethal courses-of-events together which bring about death in visible association with the structural or functional failure or inadequacy of the same general organ system. The cause of this failure or inadequacy may be anything whatever in the whole range of pathology. It may be due to lack of resistance to bacterial infections; it may be due to trophic disturbances; it may be due to mechanical alterations preventing the continuance of normal functions; or to any other cause whatever. The basis of this classification, in short, is not pathological causation, but relative biological organ-worth; relative ability to maintain its part in the structural and functional integrity of the whole organism (eucrasia), on the one side, and to resist the influence of harmful agents on the other. This classification looks at death from a purely biological rather than a medical standpoint. What part of the organism is it that, not being able to continue to function, brings about death in a particular case and a particular disease?

This question implies a significant point. The normal integrated functioning (eucrasia) of the healthy living individual is something pertaining to the organism as a whole ; the dyscrasia which is disease begins, on the other hand, at some particular locality, in a particular tissue, organ, or organ system. The organism, in short, lives as a whole, but dies piecemeal. The whole can survive no longer than the eventual failure of its weakest or poorest part. The picture revealed at the vast majority of autopsies is of many tissues and organs of the body in a quite normal state (or if abnormal so slightly affected as not to have interfered significantly with continued functioning if all else had been well) and only one or at most a few organs with such serious lesions as to have made further functioning impossible. This is, of course, the underlying biological reason for the usefulness of surgery. An organ begins to break down ; the surgeon removes the failing part and by so doing enables the whole organism to keep on living. An acute appendix furnishes a dramatic example precisely to the point. The individual as a whole may be perfectly healthy, but the breakdown of the appendix kills him if the surgeon does not get it out promptly enough.

The philosophy of the organological classification finds its roots in some part in the fruitful idea advanced by Wilhelm Roux, at about the turn of the century, to the effect that in the embryonic development of organisms there was going on all the time a struggle between the parts for advantages in nourishment, position, and all other biological goods. Certain of the consequences of this idea were taken over into medicine, particularly psychiatry, by Adler,[9] who clearly perceived the importance attendant upon different degrees of innate biological ' worth ' or value in organ systems and organs.

The idea of relative biological organworth has lately been taken up by Streeter[10] from the embryological standpoint, but without any reference to its long history or to the considerable body of research which has been devoted to it by other workers. He says (pp. 3-4) : " Our body is not like the Deacon's masterpiece that went to pieces ' all at once, and nothing first.' We are more like the automobile, made of materials of unequal durability, necessitating discard while much of it is still strong and intact. The outskirts of our cities are marred by

24

automobile graveyards, great disorderly piles of entangled relics of relatively good iron and steel. Similarly in the autopsy room we see human mechanisms which are wrecked only because of injury or defect of some single critical organ system, for the loss of which the body could not compensate. In less serious things the unequal endurance of our various tissues is a matter of common observation. We take it for granted that our teeth are going to yield to decay early. We expect presbyopia at 50 years. In many individuals the hair follicles of the scalp, normal enough in earlier years, succumb prematurely, with genetic precision, in spite of the most desperate efforts to preserve them. In other families there is poor survival power of the mechanism that provides capillary pigment, and the members find their hair streaked with gray in early adult life. On the other hand some of our tissues are super-tissues which do their work easily without sign of wearing out. The skeletal muscles appear to be adequate for a much greater life span than ours, and it would appear possible that such tissues as have the

25

power of self-replacement might go on indefinitely."

Pende[29], in his important treatise on inadequacies of constitution, devotes the second volume to the discussion of the defects, abnormalities, and inadequacies peculiar to each of the several organ systems, giving a separate chapter to each. From this discussion an excellent idea may be gained of the great variety of factors that may be involved in the determination of different biological organ worth.

A considerable number of investigations have been made in my laboratory and elsewhere[11] with the help of the organological classification of diseases and causes of death. What has it taught us about constitution in relation to disease that was not well understood before? I think that the following points may fairly be listed in answer to this question :

1. That different organ systems appear to possess inherently widely different innate biological (constitutional) worths, and are consequently associated with widely different proportions of the totals of human mortality. Generally speaking the respiratory system appears to be man's

constitutionally weakest organ system, having regard to the physiological demands upon it, and its ability to resist harmful agents and influences.

2. That there appear to be smaller, but still significant differences between races (in so far as may be judged by comparison of whites with negroes) in respect of the biological (constitutional) worth or value of their several organ systems.[12]

3. That there has been and is presumably still going on, in the series of vertebrate animals from reptiles through birds and mammals to and including man, what appears to be a progressive evolutionary change in the innate biological (constitutional) worth or value of certain organ systems.[13] This change may be most clearly perceived in the case of the nervous system, where the general biological rule that a price must always be paid for extreme specialization appears to hold. Thus while the central nervous system has become progressively a better integrative organ in the course of its evolution,[14] it seems to have weakened constitutionally in the process, in the sense that it breaks down more frequently, in such manner as to lead to the death of the

organism. Its resistance to infectious agents seems to have weakened as its complexity has increased. The same thing appears to be true of the circulatory system, though here the interpretation of the data is not quite so clear. The student of the constitutional pathology of the nervous system and of the circulatory system has before him a biological problem of much interest and potential practical importance. The increase during the last quarter of a century in the incidence of such diseases as poliomyelitis and encephalitis is worth pondering over from this point of view.

Besides these three points just discussed the organological classification of disease has led to another tentative generalization or synthesis of hitherto scattered observations, which I should like now to discuss briefly. Once the various diseases and causes of death have been sorted out by this classification it becomes possible to regroup them in such manner as to test various ideas or hypotheses. One of such possible rearrangements[15] is based on the obvious truism that the structural organization of the vertebrate body is such that certain organ systems come normally and regularly into direct and immediate contact with the external environment, while other organ systems do not, but are on the contrary protected from such contact. On this basis the organ systems may be classified as follows:

A. Organ systems coming into direct contact with the external environment	B. Organ systems not coming into direct contact with the external environment
Respiratory system	Circulatory system
Sex organs	Skeletal and muscular system
Kidneys and associated excretory organs	Nervous system
Alimentary tract	Endocrine system
Skin	

Little comment on this arrangement is necessary. The respiratory system and the alimentary tract are obviously in direct contact with environmental materials all the time. The primary and secondary sex organs are either directly exposed to environmental influences, or are directly accessible with greater or less ease to infectious agents from the environment through ducts or tubes. Even the breasts are subject to infection from external sources through the ducts of the nipples.

On the other hand the organ systems in column B present a different picture. The circulatory system is a wholly internal closed system which nowhere comes *directly* into contact with the external world under normal circumstances. The same is true of the skeleton and muscles. Certain of the latter, to be sure, have only the skin as protection against external traumatic injury, but still it remains true that everywhere there is something (skin or mucous membrane) between muscles and the external world. These tissues when in their normal unbroken state are a rather highly effective protective mechanism against infection from external sources. The central nervous system is obviously well protected against direct contact with the external environment. The thyroid, pituitary, and adrenal glands, and the islands of Langerhans are normally never in contact with, nor accessible to direct contact with the external environment.

Arranging the causes of death acccording to this A and B scheme leads at once to the following generalization : With advancing adult age the proportion of deaths due to causes having their pathological lesions or clinical manifestations associated with the organ systems of the body which are normally and regularly in direct contact with the external environment *decreases*.

On the other hand the proportion having their pathological lesions or clinical manifestations associated with the organ systems normally protected from direct contact with - the external environment *increases* as age advances.

This is shown graphically in Fig. 1.

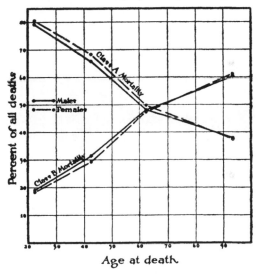

FIG. 1. The trends, at four adult age periods from age 20-24 on to the end of the life span, of mortality having its pathological lesions and/or clinical manifestations associated with (A) organ systems normally in direct contact with the external environment (plus external causes except suicide) ; and (B) organ systems normally not in direct contact with the external environment (plus ' senility ').

31

It is plain, I think, that in general the diseases usually regarded as primarily, or to a marked degree, constitutional in their etiology fall predominantly in Class B. It thus appears, from a different angle, not unreasonable that persons who attain great longevity should commonly be said to have ' sound constitutions '. They are so constructed as to be relatively immune or highly resistant to the infections and other environmental impacts, and consequently survive long ; to be taken off in the end by the wearing out and ultimate breakdown of organ systems of inherently great constitutional worth.

III

CONSTITUTION

We have so far been discoursing about constitution ' with a certain glibness. But what do we really mean, or think we mean, by this word ? To attempt to give a precise and comprehensive answer to this question would lead to the listing and discussion of a great variety of ideas that have been held upon the subject by many people. For the fact is that the concept of constitution, as relating to a living organism is an extremely complex abstraction. Even simple abstractions have a way of appearing to mean different things to different people. It will not surprise us then that the ' constitution ' of an organism appears, on the record, to have nearly if not quite as many meanings, or shades of meaning, as the number of persons who have written about it.[16]

Without attempting to review here all these different conceptions of constitution, particularly since this has been so well and so recently done by Günther, it may be said that in general they fall without great strain into two broad categories, that are in some part antithetical. The first of these includes those viewpoints which conceive constitution to mean the total make-up, status, or personality of the individual. Let us call this the *totality* view of constitution, simply for convenience in discussion. " Jeder Organismus hat eine *besondere* Konstitution ; kein Organismus ist dem anderen völlig gleich." The total personality may obviously be regarded from various points of view, leading in effect to subdivisions into so-called ' panels ', such as the morphological, the psychological, and so on. This totality concept of constitution is plainly somewhat closely related to the Aristotelian idea of ' organization '. It implies that while a man's constitution is relatively stable because heredity plays a great part in its determination, it is not something absolutely constant throughout his life. On the contrary, on this view, the constitution of an individual at any given moment is in part the resultant of his past history— the diseases he has had, the vicissitudes of embryonic development through which he passed, and so on.

The evidence that a man's biological constitution may change fundamentally during his lifetime is abundant and convincing. Consider, for example, a man who has smallpox in his thirties, and recovers from the illness. He may go on living until he is ninety. But during this long period he is immune to smallpox. He may make intimate contact with the most virulent cases of active smallpox and suffer no harm. As a result of having had the disease once he has, as an individual, undergone a profound and irreversible alteration of his biological make-up. And if this specific immunity so acquired is not to be thought of as properly a part of his constitution it would seem best to stop talking about constitution at all. If an individual were known to be born with such a complete immunity to smallpox (as presumably some people are) no one would hesitate to call it a truly constitutional peculiarity of that individual. What warrant biologically is there for regarding it as less so when it is acquired ? I know of none.

On this totality view of constitution it is the combined interaction of hereditary and environmental factors which determines the *Besonderheiten* of the differences between individual organisms. The visible, realized characteristics (phenotype) are the expression of the inherited foundation (genotype) modified and altered variously by environmental forces, acting during development primarily, but also in some degree throughout the duration of the life of the individual. The phenotypic appearance of the individual gives no sure indication as to the origin of any particular peculiarity. The work of Stockard,[17] and other experimental embryologists, has shown that structural peculiarities of the individual which phenotypically give the appearance of being genetically determined, are really in many cases due to alterations of normal development, particularly to differential alterations in the rate of development. In a similar way recent work[18] has shown that mental abnormalities and peculiarities of a sort usually regarded in former times as genetically determined are not infrequently merely the resultants of injuries at birth—consequences of the difficulties of getting a large head through a small pelvic outlet.

In sum, an individual's constitution is what he *is*, the totality of his particular individual being biologically considered, without particular immediate concern as to how it came to be what it is.

In some contrast to this view of constitution is the second concept to which reference has been made. Let us, again for convenience in discussion, call this the *genetic* view of constitution. This second concept stems from the notion of an elemental and mutually exclusive contrast between heredity and environment—nature and nurture. On this view the term constitution is to be restricted to that part only of a man's make-up which is determined and controlled by heredity—what is entailed and transmissible to his offspring—in distinction from what he acquires by education, infection, or any other environmental buffetings. Constitution looked at this way, is, in short, *genetic* constitution *et praeterea nihil*, determined solely by entailed ancestral genes, and therefore irrevocably fixed and without possibility of change except by gene mutations or accidents of meiosis.

Individual biological history can have no influence upon constitution, on this view; it will be the same at ninety as it was at nine, or at any other point during his life.

This view of constitution shares the advantages and disadvantages of current genetic doctrine. It rests upon a precise, specific, and mechanistic theory of heredity. In the theoretically best case it can put forward as the *vera causa* of a particular disease a specific gene, to match on equal footing the specific micro-organism of the bacteriologist as the causal agent of another particular disease. As Mr. Edmund Sparkler was accustomed to say of the ladies he esteemed, there is " no biggodd nonsense " about this way of looking at constitution. It is neat and tight. And the sort of usefulness it is capable of is attested by the following statement, made a short time ago in a scientific journal of extreme respectability. An eminent American biologist in discussing the personality of another distinguished biologist lately deceased, speaks of " the maternal genes of industry and unconquerable devotion from his peasant mother." It can only be regarded as a pity that he failed to note the *locus* of the gene for "unconquerable devotion" on a chromosome map. The genic mechanisms of such complex matters as insanity, poverty, and crime, if not entirely well understood, have at least been spread upon the record, as the phrase goes, and are available for higher syntheses by the forward-looking student of human constitution.

But, on the other hand, the philosophical constitutionalist is likely to be fretted by some of the debit items standing against the theory of the gene. It is an atomistic or 'particleist'[19] doctrine and entails adherence to the hoary nonsense of preformation. To be sure, the protagonists of the theory of the gene maintain strenuously that they are really pure in heart, about preformation. But their arguments fall short of convincing such considerable critics as Russell,[20] and Ritter,[21] for example. If genes are conceived of as material particles of finite though small size, then either the mutant gene vestigial in the chromosome of the fertilized egg (and prior to the act of fertilization in the chromosome of the germ cell) of *Drosophila* has something *specifically* to do with the appearance of vestigial wings on the imago which develops from the fertilized egg cell, or it doesn't. If it does, the doctrine is implicitly a doctrine of preformation. If it doesn't, what price would a prudent Scot offer for the whole gene theory?

It will be seen that the concept of constitution, whether the totality view or the genetic is adopted, is really a concept of contrast. Its center or focus of interest is the individual living organism, and it seeks to contrast the relatively stable elements of the organism with those which alter under the influence of the ever-changing external environment. The contrast actually made differs in the two views of constitution we have discussed. On the totality view the contrast is between two concrete, objective realities, the whole organism as it exists at a given moment, on the one hand, and the whole environment external to the organism on the other. On the genetic view the contrast is rather between two abstractions, heredity and environment as causal agents. ' Heredity ' is the abstraction constructed from the simple, ancient and universal observation that individuals standing in the relation we call close kinship to each other, are, statistically speaking, more like each other than they are like persons not standing in close kinship relation to them. ' Heredity ' is an example of a common type of human behaviour in respect of the use of words : we give to an observed phenomenon a name for purely descriptive purposes. In due time this word takes on an unexpressed but none the less definite connotation of explanation. In short, children that we are, we are always trying to sneak in a ' why ', when all we really know is ' how '. Thus in the present case the observed likeness between kin is commonly regarded as *due to* or *caused by* ' heredity '. Indeed, to express just this idea has come to be the principal reason for the existence of the word. But ' heredity ' is really only a brief description of a phenomenon, not an explanation of it. Similarly ' environment ', when used as the antonym to ' heredity ', is an abstraction. Its connotation in the present connection is that those conditions or states of the organism not due to ' heredity ' are due to or caused by ' environment '.

It has seemed to me that one's ideas about the meaning of biological constitution are helped towards clarification by a consideration of the operational[22] side of the matter. What do we actually do when we set out to form an idea of a particular individual's biological constitution ? In the present state of our knowledge of doing within this particular sphere, there are two, and only two, *kinds* of things we can do to acquire a knowledge of John Smith's constitution. These are :

(*a*) We can, at a given moment of time, observe and measure John Smith. These observations and measurements may be physical, chemical, or ' mental '. We can get his anatomical, physiological, biochemical, psychological, emotional, and other sorts of dimensions and reactions. When this has been done we shall have, with greater or less detail and elaboration as the case may be, a body of precise information as to the biological status of John Smith *at the moment when the observing and measuring was done*, and only that. Whatever inferences we may draw about his status at other times in his life history are inferences and nothing else.

(*b*) We theoretically can do the same thing as in (*a*) to certain other individuals standing in definite biological relationship

42

to John Smith, and particularly in the relation of *kinship*, that is to say, for example, to John Smith's children, if any and if catchable, or his parents, if available. If this is done we shall have a body of information which will not only be precise in respect of the children at the moment of examination, but also of a sort to make it possible to draw some inferences as to what John Smith's biological status was at the particular moment when he engendered each child observed and measured. This is so because at the moment of his genesis as an individual a definite and considerable fraction (in theory one-half) of all that John Smith, Jr. was at that moment had been an integral part of the individual we call his father, John Smith, Sr., up to that time.[23]

In short, knowledge of the constitution of an individual is derivable directly from measurement of the individual, and indirectly from measurement of his kin.

Since these are the only kinds of operations that can be performed that will furnish precise information about biological constitution, and since the only additional thing that can possibly be done is to repeat either (*a*), or (*b*), or both, a

43

number of times, the number of such times being obviously limited practically, we perceive that the only precise knowledge that can possibly be acquired regarding the constitution of a man is really derived from an examination of momentary[24] states of his being. This is as true in principle regarding those things in his make-up which are charged to heredity as it is of those consequent upon last week's environmental stresses. In fact, the point is doubly true on the hereditary side, because genetics is an indirect science, operationally considered. No one has seen, or measured, either a gene or the genotype directly. Such knowledge as we have of genes is derived by inference from operational procedures upon the phenotype (soma, chromosomes, etc.). But these operational procedures upon the soma are precisely our (*a*) and (*b*) above, in principle.

It is necessary to digress for a moment at this point to discuss a possible objection to the above operational statement. It might be alleged that a third kind of operation should be included, consisting of the keeping of John Smith *continuously* under a kind of general, non-metrical observation over long periods of time, or even theoretically for as long as he lived. Actually this is about what the general experience of mankind with itself has in fact done. But this is a fundamentally different kind of thing than the operations subsumed under (*a*) and (*b*) above, which alone give us all the precise information we can acquire about the biological status or constitution of an individual, John Smith. The only kind of ' continuous ' observation we have or can have gives us, instead of precise information, merely a vague, unprecise, and, as the continuing advances in biological, biochemical and other sorts of knowledge show, an often inaccurate basis for making inferences as to whether John Smith is or is not changing biologically with the passage of time. To get really precise information on this important question of change it will always be necessary to come back to operation (*a*) and perform it repeatedly, at measured time intervals.

To retrieve now the main thread of the argument, if it is true that whatever precise information we may be able to acquire as to an individual's constitution is derived only from examination of momentary states of his being, it plainly becomes important to see what circumstances and conditions influence these momentary states. The chart shown as Fig. 2, puts in condensed form some, at least, of the causal factors involved.

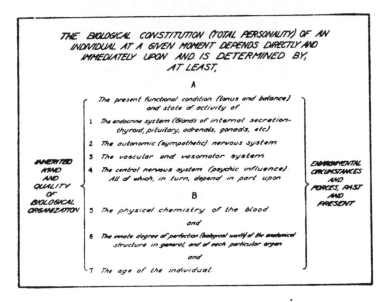

This chart, incomplete as it is, serves to make plain two things of considerable importance in thinking about constitution. One is that the making of a quantitative and comprehensive appraisal of the constitutional status or make-up of an individual is far from the simple matter that some of the current discussion of the subject would seem to imply. Too many variables are involved to leave any simplicity in the matter. The second point is that the more carefully and accurately the measurements or observations comprised in a constitutional examination are carried out the more certain it will be that the results will be of an ephemeral character, since they pertain only to the conditions at a particular moment, and since it is well known that many of the factors listed in the chart of Fig. 2 vary considerably in time, for any given individual.

As a matter of fact the material and functional status of an individual changes enormously and in diverse ways in the course of his lifetime. These changes have constituted a major problem for philosophers, biological and other, for a long time. Samuel Butler[25] presents the difficulty in the following words (pp. 78 and 79) :

"We regard our personality as a simple definite whole ; as a plain, palpable, individual thing, which can be seen going about the streets

47

or sitting indoors at home, which lasts us our lifetime, and about the confines of which no doubt can exist in the minds of reasonable people. But in truth this ' we ', which looks so simple and definite, is a nebulous and indefinable aggregation of many component parts which war not a little among themselves, our perception of our existence at all being perhaps due to this very clash of warfare, as our sense of sound and light is due to the jarring of vibrations. Moreover, as the component parts of our identity change from moment to moment, our personality becomes a thing dependent upon time present, which has no logical existence, but lives only upon the sufferance of times past and future, slipping out of our hands into the domain of one or other of these two claimants the moment we try to apprehend it. And not only is our personality as fleeting as the present moment, but the parts which compose it blend some of them so imperceptibly into, and are so inextricably linked on to, outside things which clearly form no part of our personality, that when we try to bring ourselves to book, and determine wherein we consist, or to draw a line as to where we begin or end, we find ourselves completely baffled. There is nothing but fusion and confusion ''.

Further on Butler says (p. 85) : " if that hazy contradiction in terms, ' personal identity ', be once allowed to retreat behind the threshold of the womb, it has eluded us once for all. What is true of one hour before birth is true of two, and so on till we get back to the impregnate ovum, which may fairly claim to have been personally identical with the man of eighty into which it ultimately developed, in spite of the fact that there is no particle of same matter nor sense of continuity between them, nor recognized community of instinct, nor indeed of anything which goes to the making up of that which we call identity ".

The great Erewhonian's only way out of the problem is (p. 81) " by the simple process of ignoring it : we decline, and very properly, to go into the question of where personality begins and ends, but assume it to be known to every one, and throw the onus of not knowing it upon the over-curious, who had better think as their neighbours do, right or wrong, or there is no knowing into what villainy they may not presently fall."

A somewhat different view of the case is afforded by Cuvier's[26] ' whirlpool ' concept of the organism, stated as follows : " La vie est donc un tourbillon plus ou moins rapide, plus ou moins compliqué, dont la direction est constante, et qui entraîne toujours des molécules de mêmes sortes, mais où les molécules individuelles entrent et d'ou elles sortent continuelle-ment, de manière que la *forme* du corps vivant lui est plus essentielle que sa *matière*."

49

Cuvier's *forme*, which is essentially the same thing as Aristotle's ' organization '[27] certainly changes less, either quantitatively or qualitatively, in the course of the individual's life than does the material of which the individual is composed, for example. Furthermore, it is plain that what the constitutionalist is striving to do by his measurements and observations is to get and record as sound a description as possible of this *forme*, or ' organization ', or ' pattern ', of the individual. That he has not so far, in my opinion, made much more than a beginning of progress in this direction will appear as we proceed. But there can be no question from a biological point of view[28] that the goal he has set for himself is the correct one. Practically, as constitutional biology and medicine develope there will be a methodical search for those measurable characters of the organism which change least with age, with environment, and under the action of the factors set forth in the chart above (Fig. 2). Such characters will, in general, be indices of innate, constitutional conditions, and presumably some that have real and considerable significance as indices may be found.

50

IV

SOMATOLOGY

In the modern recrudescence of interest in the constitutional element in medicine *somatology* (bodily habitus) as an index of constitution has taken the center of the stage. A number of medical men[29] have sought to find out whether there is a significant relationship between human form and human nature. To this end the external form of the human body has been more carefully re-studied, with the help of the exact methods of physical anthropology and the stimulus of some new ideas.

The principal outcome of this renewed activity has been a two-fold one ; various attempted classifications of all somatological variations into a few broad categories, called types, of bodily habitus ; and the bringing forward of some statistical and a great deal more clinical evidence tending to show some differential association of certain disease types with certain bodily habitus types.

The biological basis of the various classifications of human bodily habitus types is found fundamentally in the fact that man is a vertebrate animal. The vertebrate plan of structure comprises a principal and primary bodily axis which is the longitudinal one, with cephalic and caudal ends. The secondary axes are two in number, and at right angles to each other, the dorso-ventral axis, and the lateral axis. The external form—somatology or bodily habitus—of such an animal is plainly bound in general to depend upon the relative or proportional growth along each of these axes. Consider fish, for example : if growth along the longitudinal axis predominates an eel-like creature results ; if, on the other hand, growth along the dorso-ventral axis is greatest we get the sunfish (*Mola*) sort of result ; while finally creatures like the anglers (*Lophius*) or the bat-fish (*Malthe*) are consequences of predominant relative growth along the lateral axis. All organisms built upon the general plan of similar primary longitudinal and secondary lateral and depth axes exhibit similar differences in bodily habitus type. For example, Wheeler[30] has given interesting

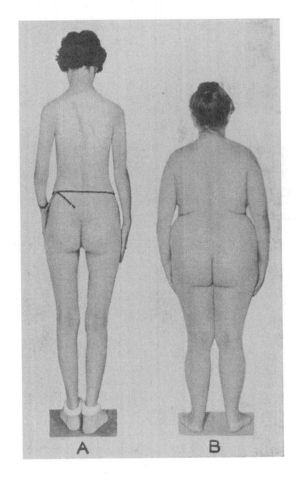

Plate I.   Rear view of two women.
A. Asthenic.   B. Pyknic.

illustrations of longitudinal and lateral bodily types in insects.

In man the two extreme bodily types are easily distinguishable. The individual in whose development growth along the primary or longitudinal bodily axis has predominated over that along the secondary axes is the *asthenic* ; he whose growth has been relatively greater along the secondary axes (lateral and dorso-ventral) than that along the primary axis is the *pyknic*. Plate I shows side by side a typical asthenic and a typical pyknic. The principal structural differences between the two are apparent. In choosing these individuals for illustration I have made no attempt to pick out the most extreme examples from our collection.

Certain of the more important measurements of the two women shown in Plate I are given in Table I.

A and B are of approximately the same age. In respect of all dimensions taken along the longitudinal (primary) axis of the body A is from 8 to 16 per cent larger than B. A is taller than B not only because her legs are longer, but because her trunk and her neck are longer. On the other hand B is larger than A in all dimensions involving the secondary axes (width and depth) of the body, by amounts ranging from 18 to more than 50 per cent. In consequence B's weight exceeds A's by 58 per cent. If we may conceive of so

TABLE 1.

Dimensions of Asthenic (A) and Pyknic (B) shown in Plate I.

Character	A	B	Percentage excess. A	B
	cm.	cm.		
Stature	163·2	145·7	+ 12·0	—
Height to ext. auditory canal	149·8	132·5	+ 13·1	—
Height to suprasternal notch	132·6	118·3	+ 12·1	—
Sitting height	86·7	80·0	+ 8·4	—
Trunk length	56·7	51·5	+ 10·1	—
Stature—Sitting height	76·5	65·7	+ 16·4	—
Head length	18·7	18·4	+ 1·6	—
Head breadth	14·3	14·2	+ 0·7	—
Head height	13·4	13·2	+ 1·5	—
Chest depth	15·9	20·1	—	+ 26·4
Chest circumference	67·9	102·0	—	+ 50·2
Neck circumference	30·0	35·5	—	+ 18·3
Circumference at umbilicus	70·8	109·0	—	+ 54·0
Body weight	45·0 kg.	71·2 kg.	—	+ 58·2

gruesome a thing as these two women being cut up into horizontal slices each 1 cm. in thickness, the average weight of A's slices would be 275 grams (9.7 ounces), while the average slice of B would weigh 489 grams (17.2 ounces).

The most lively and penetrating, and at the same time comprehensive description in concise form of the salient characteristics of asthenics and pyknics known to me is that given by Wheeler (*loc. cit.*, p. 2) and with his permission I quote it here :

" The asthenic is pale, scrawny, long-limbed, with narrow head and face (' hatchet-faced '), long, narrow, straight nose, small, often receding chin, narrow chest and abdomen, deficient development of fat and musculature, reduced pilosity on the body but often with abundant cranial thatch, abstemious, dyspeptic, with a tendency to tuberculosis, and when insane, schizophrenic, i.e., prone to fixed ideas, ideas of persecution, etc. This type is active, intense, intellectual, self-centered (introverted), often deficient in a sense of humor, fond of reforming, dogmatic or fanatical, and not infrequently detestable when claiming a too intimate knowledge of the Almighty's plans for making the world safe for democracy. The pycnic—so called, not because he likes picnics, though no other type is so fond of them—but from the Greek word πυκνός, meaning compact or thickset—is rubicund, rotund. large-bodied, short-limbed, broad through the chest, but broader through the abdomen, with round or pentagonal face, pug or thick nose, moderately pilose, fond of eating and drinking, eupeptic, with a tendency to apoplexy and arteriosclerosis ; on the mental side cyclothymic, i.e., predisposed to the recurring, circular or manic-depressive forms of insanity, such as melancholia ; extroverted, socially easy-going, tolerant in morals and religion and often very lovable because claiming no inside information in regard to the Almighty's designs ".

These two types, the asthenic and pyknic, represent the two extreme results of differential relative growth along the primary and secondary bodily axes. Being extreme variants they are relatively rare, as compared with the great number of intermediate forms lying between them. Some students of constitution have designated by special terms, such as ' athletic ', ' muscular type ', ' normal ', ' eumorphic ', etc. those individuals who are neither asthenic nor pyknic but roughly halfway between the two. This seems ill advised. Actually there is a continuous gradation by indefinitely minute steps from the extreme asthenic to the extreme pyknic habit of body. There is nowhere any discontinuity, nothing upon which to base a definite segregation into real types. The individuals who are not asthenics or pyknics are simply individuals in whose development there has been a more even balancing of growth potentials relative to the primary and secondary axes of the body.[31]

It may help to an understanding of the matter to examine Fig. 3, designed to illustrate the point. At the two ends of a bar are boxes containing double-headed arrows to indicate the direction of predominant growth, the vertical arrow

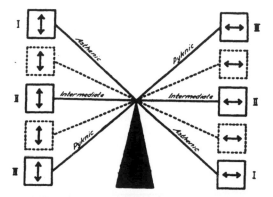

Fig. 3. Diagram to illustrate the biological conception of bodily habitus. Explanation in text.

meaning longitudinal and the horizontal arrow lateral growth. In the position I-I of the bar, with the vertical arrow in a position of maximal ascendancy, we have the condition representing the typical asthenic. Now consider the bar to swing to the position III-III. Here the horizontal arrow is at the top, and we have the typical pyknic. The bar may take any position between I-I and III-III, as indicated by the dotted bars. In so doing it will represent the bodily habitus of component units of the majority of human beings, intermediate between asthenics and

57

pyknics, some being nearer to the one than the other, and some exactly half-way between. These latter are the perfect intermediates, II-II of the diagram. Our experience in typing human beings indicates that the number of positions that the bar may (and does) take between I-I and III-III is indefinitely large. In other words the variation is continuous. Our observations lead unequivocally to the same conclusion that was reached by Wertheimer and Hesketh[39] (p. 71) : " there are no types in the strict sense, but only transitions which fit into a normal frequency curve, the extreme forms impressing one as types."

A few illustrations (Plates II-IV inclusive) will perhaps make clearer in another way some of the implications and consequences of differential relative growth along the primary and secondary axes of the body. In all of these plates the scale of reduction from the original is identical, and the same as in Plate I. The general scheme upon which these illustrations have been made is to alter photographically certain measurements of either individual A or individual B of Plate I so that they will be identical with the same

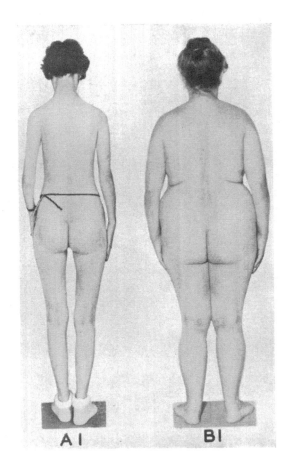

Plate II. A 1 = A (Plate I). B 1 = B enlarged
to the same total height as A.

measurements in the other, at the same time preserving all the *proportions* of their bodily make-up exactly as they were before the alteration of the particular measurement. Thus in Plate II, the total height of the pyknic individual (B) has been made equal to the total height of the asthenic individual (A). B1 of Plate II shows this altered individual alongside the unaltered A. While increasing B's stature to that shown in B 1 we have at the same time increased all her other bodily dimensions in exactly the same proportion. Plate II then shows graphically the answer to the following question : supposing that B had grown along the *longitudinal* axis of the body *absolutely* as much as A actually did, but had at the same time preserved the same proportion between her (B's) lateral and longitudinal growth that she did in her actual development, how then would she have compared in appearance with A ?

Suppose we next make B's *legs* as long as A's, keeping all of B's dimensions in the same proportions that they have in actual fact. The result is shown in Plate III.

We see that if B were enlarged all round, keeping her actual natural proportions, up to the point where her *legs* were absolutely of the same length as A's she would then be half a head taller than A, and altogether a large woman.

Let us next reduce B to the point where she will have exactly the same *chest breadth* as A, preserving her natural proportions as before. Plate IV shows the result.

Plainly if B had grown *laterally* to the same absolute degree as A, and at the same time preserved her actual natural proportions, she would have been rather tiny — a sort of pygmy pyknic—standing only about 115 cm. (45.3 inches) tall.

While attention has so far been focussed upon differential growth in the discussion of the differences between asthenics and pyknics it is not to be inferred that this is the only thing involved in the case biologically. Asthenics and pyknics differ in other respects beside bodily habitus. The point it seems desirable to emphasize is that the observable differences in external bodily form between these two kinds of individuals are the direct and immediate consequences of differential relative growth along the primary and secondary axes of the body. What lies

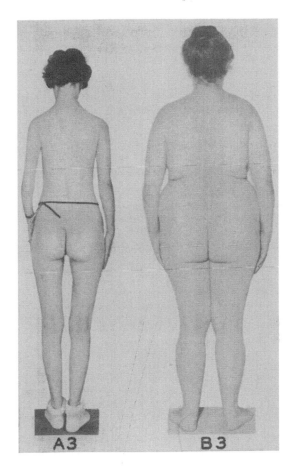

Plate III. A 3 = A (Plate I). B 3 = B enlarged
to have the same leg length as A.

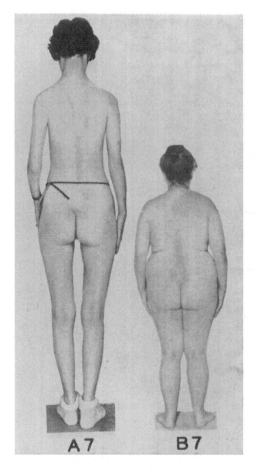

Plate IV.   A 7 = A (Plate I).   B 7 = B reduced
to the same chest breadth as A.

behind and determines these differentials in relative growth, and what correlated phenomena go along with them in other departments of the general biological economy, are other and different problems lying outside the field of immediate discussion. It is known that differences in the functioning of certain endocrine organs influence profoundly the growth differentials under discussion.[32] Also it is certain that inheritance plays a great rôle in determining whether a particular individual shall be of the preponderantly longitudinal or the preponderantly lateral habit of growth. That this is so is a matter of simple observation to everyone. Bodily habitus " runs in families " as the phrase goes. Consider, for example, such a family as the Bogues, a family which certainly exemplifies the first line of Goethe's
    " Vom Vater hab' ich die Statur,
        Des Lebens ernstes Führen."
The reported facts about this family,[33] are as follows : Hiram Bogue, a man 7 feet tall, married a woman 5 ft. 10 inches in height. Ten children from the union grew up, in both the literal and figurative senses of the words. Their heights were as follows : Ray (6 ft. 7 ins.) ; Glenna (6 ft.) ;

Anna (6 ft.) ; Max (7 ft. 2 ins.) ; Arthur. (6 ft. 6.5 ins.) ; Homer (6 ft. 6 ins.) ; Howard (6 ft. 6 ins.) ; Alvin (6 ft. 7 ins.) ; Lelant (6 ft. 8 ins.) ; Ida (6 ft.). Here are ten siblings, the closest of kin, all six feet or more in height whether male or female. Some impression of how far this family deviates from a random sample of human beings in general, in respect of preponderant growth along the primary longitudinal axis of the body, may be gained by contrasting their 100 per cent achievement of six feet and over with the fact that among Scottish recruits (all males naturally) only about 3.6 per cent.[34] are six-footers or better. And the Scots are among the tallest of modern peoples, as a racial group. This Bogue family is, of course, only a single striking example. That inheritance plays a major rôle in the determination of bodily habitus generally was first demonstrated by Galton,[35] confirmed and extended by Pearson and Lee,[36] and brought into direct relation to present-day constitutional studies by Davenport.[37]

Up to this point the discussion has been of the so-called ' pure types ' of bodily

habitus, the asthenics, pyknics, and intermediates. But one of the first observations
to emerge from a systematic study of the
body build of human beings is that all of
them cannot be successfully put into these
' pure ' pigeon-holes, however determined
the observer may be to dispose of them so.
The reason is a simple one. Some
individuals are so constructed that while
certain parts of their bodies fall plainly
into the asthenic category, other parts are
quite as clearly pyknic in their form. Such
individuals, in short, are *mixtures* or
mosaics in their morphology. The term
which has come to be generally used in
the literature of somatology to designate
this sort of bodily habitus is *dysplastic*
(and for the biological phenomenon giving
rise to such types, *dysplasia* or
dysplasticity), in contrast to *euplastic*. The
dysplastic individual is envisioned, by this
terminology, as badly moulded or formed,
because his bodily proportions (*a*) depart
from our ideals for the human form, and
(*b*) are inconsistent among themselves.
The euplastic individual, *par excellence*, is
the exact intermediate between the typical
asthenic and the typical pyknic, and
represents the aesthetic ideals regarding

the human form which our civilization has derived by social and cultural inheritance from the Greeks of the time of Pericles.[38] The euplastic is the well-formed person, symmetrically and consistently put together. He may be asthenic or pyknic, but in each case he must be consistent to his type in all his parts.

Two examples of dysplasticity in human form are shown in Plate V.

It will be seen from Plate V that individual X has the trunk of an extreme asthenic supported upon the legs of a pyknic. Individual Y, on the other hand, has the trunk of a pyknic and the limbs of an asthenic. Neither X nor Y would be regarded as beautiful.

Examination of large numbers of individuals demonstrates at once that dysplasticity is itself a graded phenomenon, a matter of continuously varying degree of departure from symmetrical proportions, as might have been expected *a priori*. The examples shown in Plate V were chosen because they illustrated the phenomenon in rather extreme and striking form. But between such odd biological architecture and the perfect symmetry of the Venus de Milo there can be found any

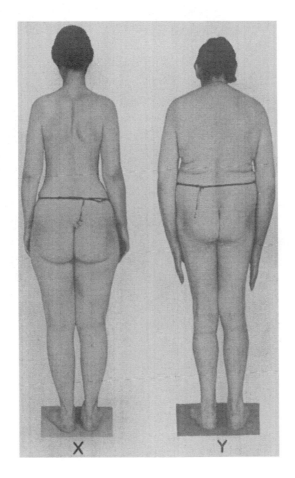

Plate V. Two dysplastic women.

number of gradations. This leads to the necessity for some sort of index of dysplasticity, simple enough to be practically usable in classifying human beings in respect of their somatology. In our constitutional work here the following scheme has been used. Individuals are graded as to trunk type and limb type separately on the scales shown in Fig. 4.

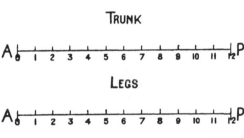

Fig. 4. Scales used in grading somatological types.

An extreme pyknic symmetrically developed, that is to say euplastic, would be checked 12/12 on the scales, meaning that in respect of both trunk and limbs this individual embodied the extreme of development in the pyknic direction. Similarly the most extreme asthenic would be checked 0/0. But a dysplastic individual might be recorded as 10/3, meaning that

C

he had a trunk well over on the pyknic side, associated with limbs definitely of the asthenic type.

In our work we have found it convenient to use as a rough index of dysplasticity the numerical difference, without regard to sign, between the two recorded scale numbers. The dysplasticity index for the individual mentioned would be $10-3 = 7$. For the perfectly euplastic individual the index will be zero, and in the most extreme case of dysplasia it cannot rise above the value of 12. In the next section of this discussion we shall have occasion to use this index of dysplasia.

The phenomenon which the modern student of constitution calls dysplasia is what lies objectively behind the old concept of ' mosaic inheritance '. Whole regions or parts of the body are sometimes observed to ' hang together ' in inheritance, and to be sharply marked off from other regions or parts in so doing. The dysplastic individual exhibits exactly this sort of thing. His appearance is as if his creator had had before him an old-fashioned type-setter's case, in the compartments of which instead of types were parts of the body—here the legs, there the arms, in the upper row the faces, just below the trunks, and so on—and in the last distribution of the type back to the case several founts had been mixed, with the result that in ' setting up ' this particular dysplastic individual the compositor had accidently picked up a pair of legs, say, of a wrong fount. The dysplastic, in short, looks like a page of bad galley before it has been proof-read.

This phenomenon of coarse mosaic inheritance is capable of at least a formal explanation in the modern chromosome theory of heredity. The hanging together in inheritance of a group of unit characters is called ' linkage ' in current genetic terminology, and is held to be due to the presence in the same chromosome of the genes of all the unit characters which hang together in their transmission from generation to generation.

V

HEALTH

It has been pointed out in earlier
sections that somatological constitutions
of particular sorts have long been known
by clinicians to be more frequently subject
to certain diseases than others. The
tuberculous person is often (but not
always) of asthenic habitus ; the asthenic
is more often tuberculous than the pyknic.
Cerebral hemorrhage occurs often (but
not always) in persons of the pyknic habit
of body ; and the pyknic is (perhaps) more
often apoplectic than the asthenic. The
few relationships of this sort between
bodily habitus and disease, while founded
upon essentially stochastic reasoning, have
not, generally speaking, been subjected to
really thorough and penetrating statistical
analysis. In particular, there has been very
little done, so far as I am aware, in the way
of an attempt to find whether persons of
a particular habitus of body, say asthenics,
or pyknics, or euplastics, or dysplastics,

enjoy generally better or worse health than those of other bodily forms.

I should like to present briefly some results of a very modest attempt to throw some light on this question.[39] On account of the relatively small numbers involved, and the intrinsic complexity and difficulty of the problem, the results can only be regarded as suggestive, and in no sense as finally conclusive. But, as every practical worker on constitution knows, to make complete and thorough constitutional examinations and records, under uniform and consistent plans and conditions, on even as many as 290 adults of the same sex and marital status, is no small task. In the nature of the case our knowledge in this field is bound to advance slowly. But the present contribution may perhaps be useful as suggesting methods of inquiry.

The following discussion is based upon the constitutional records of 290 white women, each of whom had been pregnant one or more times.[40] All but seven of them were married. Their case histories form a part of the general collection of constitutional records in the archives of the Department of Biology of the School of Hygiene and Public Health of the Johns

69

Hopkins University. The methods used in the collecting of these records have been fully described elsewhere[41] and need not be repeated here.

Table 2 shows the distribution of these 290 women relative to three variables, viz., age, bodily habitus, and general health up to the time of record. The first of these variables is self-explanatory. Regarding the second, it should be said that trunk habitus and limb habitus are separately tabulated, and that *asthenic* is defined as anything falling in the range 0—3 (inclusive) of our typing scale (*vide supra*) ; *intermediate* as anything falling in the range 4—8 (inclusive) ; and *pyknic* as anything between 9 and 12 (inclusive) on the same scale.

The records of health refer to each subject's general health during her lifetime up to the time of our record, that is to say until she was given the constitutional examination. The health records are graded according to the following scale, which we have used with satisfactory results in earlier investigations :

V.G. = Very good (never ill)
G. = Good (minor ailments only)
F. = Fair (average amount of sickness)
P. = Poor (frequently sick)
V.P. = Very poor (an invalid throughout life)

70

In the present group no individual fell in the V.P. class. For purposes of tabulation we have grouped the V.G.'s and the G.'s together in a single class.

From Table 2 we note, considering first the totals for all ages together that :

1. The distribution of habitus type is substantially similar whether the typing is based on trunk alone or on limbs alone. In round terms, a fifth or fewer of these women were of the asthenic habitus ; a shade under a quarter of them were of the pyknic habitus ; and the remainder, somewhat more than half, were in the intermediate group in respect of habitus. Closer examination of the figures shows that typing on the basis of the limbs alone throws fewer into the extreme types (asthenic and pyknic) and more into the intermediate type, as compared with the typing on the basis of trunk alone.

2. The general health of these women throughout their lives up to the time of the examination had, on the whole, been excellent. Taking all ages and all habitus types together 78.6 per cent fell in the combined class of ' Very good ' and ' Good ', and 13.1 per cent in the class ' Fair ', leaving only 8.3 per cent of the

71

TABLE 2.

Age and somatological type (habitus) for trunk and limbs separately, at the time of examination, and general health prior to time of examination, for 290 white women.

Age class	General health	Asthenic (0-3) Trunk	Limbs	Intermediate (4-8) Trunk	Limbs	Pyknic (9-12) Trunk	Limbs	Totals as to health Trunk	Limbs	Per cents as to health Trunk	Limbs
Under 20	V.G.&G.	2	0	2	4	0	0	4	4	100·0	100·0
	F.	0	0	0	0	0	0	0	0	0	0
	P.	0	0	0	0	0	0	0	0	0	0
Sub-totals (under 20) as to habitus.	All healths	2	0	2	4	0	0	4	4	100	100
Per cents (under 20) as to habitus.		50·0	0	50·0	100·0	0	0	100	100	—	—
20-29	V.G.&G.	12	9	14	17	4	4	30	30	83·3	83·3
	F.	1	0	2	3	0	0	3	3	8·3	8·3
	P.	0	0	3	3	0	0	3	3	8·3	8·3
Sub-totals (20-29) as to habitus.	All healths	13	9	19	23	4	4	36	36	100	100
Per cents (20-29) as to habitus.		36·1	25·0	52·8	63·9	11·1	11·1	100	100	—	—
30-39	V.G.&G.	9	5	21	22	12	15	42	42	71·2	71·2
	F.	2	1	5	5	3	4	10	10	16·9	16·9
	P.	2	2	3	3	2	2	7	7	11·9	11·9
Sub-totals (30-39) as to habitus.	All healths	13	8	29	30	17	21	59	59	100	100
Per cents (30-39) as to habitus.		22·0	13·6	49·2	50·9	28·8	35·6	100	100	—	—
40-49	V.G.&G.	13	11	29	40	26	17	68	68	81·9	81·9
	F.	3	3	6	8	3	1	12	12	14·5	14·5
	P.	0	0	1	1	2	2	3	3	3·6	3·6

Sub-totals (40-49) as to habitus.	All healths	16	14	36	49	31	20	85	85	100	100
Per cents (40-49) as to habitus.		19·3	16·9	43·4	59·0	37·4	24·1	100	100	—	—
50-59	V.G.&G.	9	9	32	30	12	14	53	53	78·0	78·0
	F.	1	1	6	6	1	1	8	8	11·8	11·8
	P.	1	1	5	5	1	1	7	7	10·3	10·3
Sub-totals (50-59) as to habitus.	All healths	11	11	43	41	14	16	68	68	100	100
Per cents (50-59) as to habitus.		16·2	16·2	63·3	60·3	20·6	23·5	100	100	—	—
60-69	V.G.&G.	1	1	23	24	3	2	27	27	77·1	77·1
	F.	0	0	3	2	1	2	4	4	11·4	11·4
	P.	0	0	3	3	1	1	4	4	11·4	11·4
Sub-totals (60-69) as to habitus.	All healths	1	1	29	29	5	5	35	35	100	100
Per cents (60-69) as to habitus.		2·9	2·9	82·8	82·8	14·3	14·3	100	100	—	—
70-79	V.G.&G.	0	0	4	4	0	0	4	4	80·0	80·0
	F.	0	0	1	1	0	0	1	1	20·0	20·0
	P.	0	0	0	0	0	0	0	0	0	0
Sub-totals (70-79) as to habitus.	All healths	0	0	5	5	0	0	5	5	100	100
Per cents. (70-79) as to habitus.		0	0	100·0	100·0	0	0	100	100	—	—
All ages together	V.G.&G.	46	35	125	141	57	52	228	228	78·6	78·6
	F.	7	5	23	25	8	8	38	38	13·1	13·1
	P.	3	3	15	15	6	6	24	24	8·3	8·3
Totals (all ages) as to habitus.	All healths	56	43	163	181	71	66	290	290	100	100
Per cents (all ages) as to habitus.		19·3	14·8	56·2	62·4	24·5	22·8	100	100	—	—

73

whole group recorded as having had ' Poor'
health. Considering the general health
relations of the different habitus types, as
indicated by the trunk habitus classification, the results, in percentages, are as
follows :

Health	Trunk Habitus		
	Asthenic	Intermediate	Pyknic
	per cent	per cent	per cent
Very Good and Good	82·1±3·5	76·7±2·2	80·3±3·2
Fair	12·5±3·0	14·1±1·8	11·3±2·5
Poor	5·4±2·0	9·2±1·5	8·4±2·2

It is evident that in this sample of
women those of intermediate trunk habitus
type had experienced slightly poorer
general health during their lives than
either the asthenics or the pyknics. Those
of asthenic trunk habitus appear to be a
little the best of the lot in respect of general
health, but by only an insignificant margin
over the pyknics. These relations are not
essentially different if the classification is
based upon limb habitus type, as the
following figures show, although the differences are less marked than when trunk
habitus is the basis of classification.

Health	Limb Habitus		
	Asthenic	Intermediate	Pyknic
	per cent	per cent	per cent
Very Good and Good	81·4±4·0	77·9±2·1	78·8±3·4
Fair	11·6±3·3	13·8±1·7	12·1±2·7
Poor	7·0±2·6	8·3±1·4	9·1±2·4

It must, however, be clearly understood that none of these differences in respect of general health in the several bodily habitus types can be regarded as significant. They are not greater, in short, than might be expected to arise in random sampling. The only conclusion that can be drawn is that, so far as this sample of 290 women is concerned, there is no sensible difference in general health between asthenics, pyknics, or intermediates, taken as classes. Differences in bodily habitus among these women have made no significant, orderly differences in general health.

3. The 290 women as a whole group had a remarkably symmetrical age distribution about their mean age (at the time of examination) of 45.35 ± 0.52 years. Their median age was 45.54 ± 0.65 years, a value obviously not significantly different from that of the mean. The standard deviation of the group in respect of age is 13.02 ± 0.36 years. There are some significant differences in respect of age between the three habitus type groups. On the basis of trunk habitus type the mean ages array themselves as follows :—

Asthenic, 39.39 ± 1.08 years ; Pyknic,

44.86 ± 0.78 years ; Intermediate 47.64±
0.73 years. The median ages for the same
groups have very nearly the same values,
and therefore need not be given. Also the
figures arrayed on the basis of limb habitus
give essentially the same results, the means
being as follows : Asthenic, 41.98 ± 1.16
years ; Pyknic, 44.55 ± 0.87 years ; Intermediate, 46.44 ± 0.70 years. It thus
appears that, in this material, the asthenic
group is definitely the youngest group, and
the group of intermediate bodily habitus
definitely the oldest, with the pyknics
falling in between. Between the ages of 20
and 70 it appears that in this sample of
women the proportion of *asthenics* tended
to *decrease* with advancing age. The
proportion of *pyknics* in this material
tended to increase with age to about 40
years, and thereafter decrease. The proportion of *intermediates* tended to decrease
from 20 years of age to about 40 and thereafter increase. The interpretation of these
results is both difficult and doubtful,
primarily for the reason that the figures
are the result of a combination of two
varying factors, *viz.*, (*a*) any actual
biological relationship which may exist
between somatological type and age, and

(*b*) the judgment of the person (or persons) doing the typing.

The matter of health in relation to bodily habitus may be approached in another way. Have the euplastic women enjoyed better or worse health than their dysplastic colleagues ? It has been alleged by some students that dysplasia, by its very nature, indicates a general lack of organic balance, and that on that account generally poor health may be expected to be associated with it. Let us see what the present material offers on the point.

In the present study we have used the difference between the trunk and the limb typing scales (*cf.* Fig. 4) as an index of dysplasticity, and called all individuals showing a scale difference between 0 and 2 inclusive *euplastic*, and all individuals with a scale difference of 3 and over *dysplastic*. Table 3 gives the distribution of the material relative to age and general health, on the basis of this classification.

From the data of Table 3 the following biometric constants relative to age are computed :

	Euplastics years	*Dysplastics* years
Mean age	45·47 ± 0·58	44·83 ± 1·15
Median age	45·61 ± 0·73	45·28 ± 1·44
Standard deviation	13·05 ± 0·41	12·91 ± ·82

77

TABLE 3.

Dysplasticity index and age at time of examination, and general health prior to examination, for 290 white women.

Age class	General health	Euplastic habitus (Index = 0-2 inclusive)	Dysplastic habitus (Index = 3-6 inclusive)	Totals as to health	Per cent. as to health
Under 20	V.G. and G.	3	1	4	100·0
	F.	0	0	0	0
	P.	0	0	0	0
Sub-totals(under 20)as to habitus.	All healths	3	1	4	100
Per cent (under 20) as to habitus.		75·0	25·0	100	—
20-29	V.G. and G.	23	7	30	83·3
	F.	2	1	3	8·3
	P.	3	0	3	8·3
Sub-totals (20-29) as to habitus.	All healths	28	8	36	100
Per cent (20-29) as to habitus.		77·8	22·2	100	—
30-39	V.G. and G.	36	6	42	71·2
	F.	8	2	10	16·9
	P.	5	2	7	11·9
Sub-totals (30-39) as to habitus.	All healths	49	10	59	100
Per cent (30-39) as to habitus.		83·1	16·9	100	—
40-49	V.G. and G.	56	12	68	81·9
	F.	6	6	12	14·5
	P.	3	0	3	3·6

Sub-totals (40-49) as to habitus.	All healths	65	18	83	100
Per cent (40-49) as to habitus.		78·3	21·7	100	—
50-59 ..	V.G. and G.	44	9	53	78·0
	F.	5	3	8	11·8
	P.	7	0	7	10·3
Sub-totals (50-59) as to habitus.	All healths	56	12	68	100
Per cent (50-59) as to habitus.		82·3	17·7	100	—
60-69 ..	V.G. and G.	22	5	27	77·1
	F.	3	1	4	11·4
	P.	2	2	4	11·4
Sub-totals (60-69) as to habitus.	All healths	27	8	35	100
Per cent (60-69) as to habitus.		77·1	22·9	100	—
70-79	V.G. and G.	4	0	4	80·0
	F.	1	0	1	20·0
	P.	0	0	0	0
Sub-totals (70-79) as to habitus.	All healths	5	0	5	100
Per cent (70-79) as to habitus.		100·0	0	100	—
All ages together	V.G. and G.	188	40	228	78·6
	F.	25	13	38	13·1
	P.	20	4	24	8·3
Totals (all ages) as to habitus.	All healths	233	57	290	100
Per cent (all ages) as to habitus.		80.3	19·7	100	—

It is at once evident that there are no significant differences between the two groups, euplastic and dysplastic, in respect of age.

The proportion of euplastics, as here defined, to dysplastics is of interest. Almost exactly four-fifths of the subjects fell in the former class and one-fifth in the latter. Whether this is to be regarded aesthetically as a satisfactory and encouraging state of affairs, or the opposite, is a matter upon which the reader may form his own opinion.

There has been an idea among constitutional students, not particularly well supported by definite quantitative evidence, that dysplasia was to be regarded as indicative of generally poorer health and less sound constitution than euplasia. This view is to some extent supported by the present data, as the following figures show :

General Health	Euplastics per cent	Dysplastics per cent	Difference	D/PE_D
Very good and good	$80 \cdot 7 \pm 1 \cdot 7$	$70 \cdot 2 \pm 4 \cdot 1$	$+10 \cdot 5 \pm 4 \cdot 4$	$+2 \cdot 4$
Fair	$10 \cdot 7 \pm 1 \cdot 4$	$22 \cdot 8 \pm 3 \cdot 8$	$-12 \cdot 1 \pm 4 \cdot 0$	$-3 \cdot 0$
Poor	$8 \cdot 6 \pm 1 \cdot 2$	$7 \cdot 0 \pm 2 \cdot 3$	$+ 1 \cdot 6 \pm 2 \cdot 6$	$+0 \cdot 6$
	$100 \cdot 0$	$100 \cdot 0$		

It appears that the euplastics here measured show a higher percentage of persons with V.G. and G. health than the dysplastics, by an amount which is probably significant statistically. On the other hand the dysplastics in the present material have a higher percentage than the euplastics of persons with F. health, again by a probably significant amount. There is no significant difference between euplastics and dysplastics in respect of relative numbers of persons with P. health.

In general, it must be said that a careful statistical examination of rather accurate, if not very extensive material, does not yield evidence of any very marked or striking association between bodily habitus and general health. If a universal scheme of eugenics were to make all mankind over into beautiful euplastics, it does not appear on the basis of present evidence that general health would be so much better than it now is as to put any considerable number of hospitals or physicians out of business. But it must be remembered that external somatology does not tell the whole story of biological constitution. It would be very dubious logic indeed to conclude

81

generally that there is little relation between constitution and health because there is only a small degree of correlation between bodily habitus types and general health, assuming the results of the preceding study to be confirmed by further investigations. All that the present data suggest is that *one group* of variables (bodily habitus) indicative of the constitutional status of the individual does not appear to be very closely related to general health.

VI

CONCLUSION

The principal general conclusion which can be drawn, as it seems to me, from a survey at the present time of the subject of biological constitution in its relation to health and disease, is that we are really only just at the beginning of some understanding of a highly complicated and equally important matter. Little if anything in the way of general principles, soundly grounded and of established validity, has yet emerged. This is as true of the methodology and philosophy of the subject as it is of its results based upon the observation of phenomena, and it is about as true of the biological as of the medical side of the case. Furthermore it appears clear that an enormous amount of spade work—observing and above all *measuring* the variation of the human organism in respect of both its structural and functional characteristics—must still be done before there can be anything properly to be called a science of constitutional medicine and pathology.

To-day there is too much of vagueness and of *Tendenz* in the whole subject. Overt or concealed and perhaps unconscious *a priori* prejudgments stand forth in the stead of that thorough and penetrating analysis with subsequent synthesis which makes a true science. Prejudices, beliefs, sentiments, and authoritarianism, in short, play too large a rôle in the field to-day. As we have seen earlier, these unscientific attitudes appear even in the basic defining concepts of the subject. Thus the genetical viewpoint would have it that genetic constitution is paramount, and that the influences of the environment belong to another universe of discourse. Again the somatological viewpoint in the field tends rather regularly to confuse correlation with causation.

The problem of constitutional medicine —indeed more than the problem, the very essence of the subject—is statistical in character. The real objective is to find out the inter-relationships between a whole series of complex variables, anatomical, physiological, psychological, and pathological, observably characterising human beings. There is only one way open to get this desired knowledge. It is the statistical way, experiment being, in the nature of the case, largely excluded. But statistics means counting and measuring. There is no short cut here. Nothing can take the place of the patient accumulation of data—measurements made with the same sort of care and thoroughness that the physicist puts into his, taken on large enough numbers so that the canons of statistical sampling are reasonably satisfied. And these measurements must include a wide range of characteristics of the human organism before anything very profound in the way of synthesis can be expected. Fine examples of the sort of basic work necessary to establish a real science of constitution are in the long series of investigations of Karl Pearson and his students and assistants in England, regarding the variation and inheritance of physical, mental, and moral characters in man, and on a less ambitious scale the work of Reed and Love[42] on army officers in this country.

When all this spade work has been done, however, the difficulties and pitfalls will not have been wholly surmounted. The correct interpretation of data relating to constitution is sometimes extraordinarily puzzling. Let me give an example in illustration of the point. Recently Dr. Takeo Imai has published[43] the results of some three years careful work in my laboratory. His problem was to determine quantitatively the intensity of inheritance from parent to offspring in respect of certain bodily dimensions of the fly *Drosophila melanogaster*. He used material of great homogeneity, genetically and in all other biological respects. The stock of flies from which he drew the animals for his experiments had been line-bred in the laboratory for many years. They were certainly vastly more homogeneous than any race or group of human beings that ever existed. Furthermore, the characters measured were dimensions of the exoskeleton, capable of much more precise determination than most of the characters of a living man. The flies were reared under the most carefully controlled conditions, to ensure constancy and uniformity of environment. The experiments were divided into three series. The parent flies in each series were reared under identical environmental conditions in every respect,

86

and all at a constant temperatue of 25°C. The offspring in one series were reared at a constant temperature of 18°C., in another series at 23°C., and in the third series at 28°C. In all other respects the environmental conditions surrounding the offspring were identical in all three series. The parents in each series were a random sample from the same homogeneous stock. After the offspring had emerged as imagoes the same bodily characteristics were measured on them as had been measured on their parents, and correlation tables between parent and offspring were formed, and correlation coefficients computed. According to the accepted canons of biometric methodology these coefficients of parent-offspring correlation measure the intensity of heredity in this kinship relationship, for the characters measured.

The net result of the study was that in the 28° series the average parent-offspring correlation for all characters measured was sensibly zero (+0.020), indicating that there was no inheritance at all. In the 23° series the average coefficient rose to +0.051, more than double the value at 28°, but still absolutely so small as to indicate no significant inheritance. But in the 18° series the coefficient had a value of +0.245, indicating a substantial intensity of inheritance, not too different from what would theoretically be expected on the basis of the statistical law of ancestral inheritance.

Now if, in these experiments, *only* the 18° temperature had been tried, the results would have appeared clear and unequivocal. The result expected *a priori* would have emerged, and one more instance would have been put upon the record as confirming and further establishing the law of ancestral inheritance. But as the actual results show, the state of intellectual satisfaction so engendered would have rested upon a poor foundation. Does not this case emphasize the need for extreme caution in drawing conclusions from statistical data in regard to the inheritance of human characters?

Although it has seemed necessary and desirable to emphasize the difficulties inherent in the investigation of human constitution, and the not altogether satisfactory state of present achievement towards an understanding of the subject, I should not like to close on this note. If there are difficulties in the subject there are also great opportunities and promise. And furthermore there is a kind of moral necessity to go forward in the attempt to get a better understanding of the whole nature of man, lest he perish. The material, mechanized civilization he has evolved may easily become a monster to destroy him unless he learns better to comprehend, develop, and control his biological nature. Somewhat belatedly it is beginning to be seen that inventions and discoveries that cannot be intelligently managed after they are made are likely to be a curse rather than a blessing. " The fact is, there has been a sad lagging behind the advance of science on the part of what may be termed the non-scientific world, that is, the ethical and spiritual, and we might add, the political. There has been no preparing of the ground for the coming of the gifts of science, and the result is that much that should otherwise have been a benefit to mankind has simply led to social chaos."[44]

The student of constitution has a major rôle to play in the development of an adequate understanding of human nature.

VII

NOTES AND REFERENCES

[1] *Cf.* Brock, A. J., *Galen on the Natural Faculties*, London and New York (Loeb Classical Library) 1916. He says (p. xii) : " As we recognize, in our popular everyday psychology, that ' it takes two to make a quarrel ', so Hippocrates recognized that in pathology, it takes two (organism and environment) to make a disease."

[2] I quote from the American reprint of Francis Adams' translation, omitting his notes on textual and other points (Adams, F., *The Genuine Works of Hippocrates*, New York, 1929).

[3] For a perfectly delightful castigation of those of his medical *confrères* who hold such views, see F. G. Crookshank's *Individual Diagnosis*. (Psyche Miniatures, Medical Series No. 13), London, 1930.

[4] Brock, *loc. cit.*, p. 197.

[5] *De motu animalium* (The Works of Aristotle translated into English) II, 703a, 30-35, Oxford, 1912.

[6] Bernard, Léon. " Tuberculose et hérédité ", *Presse Médicale*, March 24, 1928.

[7] For an interesting discussion of this treatise, see Egdahl, A., " Linnaeus' ' Genera Morborum ', and some of his other medical works ", *Med. Lib. and Hist. Jour.*, Vol. 5, pp. 185-193, 1907.

[8] Pearl, R., " Certain evolutionary aspects of human mortality rates ", *Amer. Nat.*, Vol. 54, pp. 5-44, 1920. This paper gives the first statement of the author's organological classification.

[9] Adler, A., *Studie über Minderwertigkeit von Organen*, München, 1927. [This is a revised reprint. The book was first published in 1907.]

Adler was the first to develop systematically the idea of differences in innate organ-worth in relation to human pathology. He rightly says (p. 4) : " Die Lehre von der Minderwertigkeit der Organe Probleme in Angriff nimmt, die zu den wichtigsten der Pathologie gehören ". But in more general terms the idea of differing innate biological worth or fitness of organ systems was implicit in Roux' discussion of the " Kampf der Teile ".

[10] Streeter, G. L. " Focal deficiencies in fetal tissues and their relation to intra-uterine amputations ", *Carnegie Inst. of Washington, Publ. No. 414, Contrib. to Embryol.*, Vol. 22, pp. 1-44, 1930.

[11] See Pearl, R., and T. Raenkham, " Studies on human longevity. V. Constitutional factors in mortality at advanced ages ", *Human Biology*, Vol. 4, pp. 80-118, 1932, for a partial list of such studies.

[12] Pearl, R., " Biological factors in negro mortality ", *Human Biology*, Vol. 1, pp. 229-249, 1929.

[13] Pearl, R., " Evolution and mortality ", *Quart. Rev. Biol.*, Vol. 3, pp. 271-280, 1928.

[14] It should be clearly understood that we are here discussing *evolutionary* changes on a long time base, and not short-period secular changes in current mortality.

[15] See Pearl and Raenkham, *loc. cit., supra.*

[16] Günther, H., " Grundprobleme der Konstitutionsforschung ", Leipzig, 1929, pp. 155-177. This constitutes Heft 3 of Band IV of the *Würzburger Abhandlungen aus der Gesamtgebiet der Medizin.*

[17] Stockard, C. R., *The Physical Basis of Personality*, New York, 1931.

[18] For a general review of this subject see *Birth Injuries of the Central Nervous System*, Part I.—Cerebral Birth Injuries, by Frank R. Ford ; Part II—Cord Birth Injuries, by Bronson Crothers and Marian C. Putnam, Baltimore, 1927. Extensive bibliographies are given there.

[19] This is a dreadful word, for which I disclaim all responsibility except that of quotation. If it is to be used at all, it ought in common decency to be written ' particle-ist ' ; but even then it will make anyone shudder who has the slightest feeling for the dignity and honor of his mother tongue.

[20] Russell, E. S., *The Interpretation of Development and Heredity. A Study in Biological Method.* Oxford, 1930.

[21] Ritter, W. E., '' Why Aristotle invented the word ' entelecheia ', '' *Quart. Rev. Biol.*, Vol. 7, pp. 377-404, 1932.

[22] In the sense that P. W. Bridgeman uses this word in his masterly treatise, *The Logic of Modern Physics*, New York, 1927.

[23] The reader who has not kept abreast of recent work on the development of the gonads and germ-cells must be prepared for something of a shock at the inroads that have been made upon the observational basis available to Weismann and relied on by him for his great generalization of an unbridgeable and eternal gap between soma and germ. An excellent recent review of this field will be found in Heys, Florence, '' The problem of the origin of germ cells '', *Quart. Rev. Biol.*, Vol. 6, pp. 1-45, 1931. This paper has an extensive bibliography. As investigation progresses the observations of the actual formation of germ-cells and their relations to the rest of the body are seen to be more and more irreconcilable with Weismann's general theory of heredity (and with other later theories similar to it in their fundamental philosophy) and more and more in accord with the organismal view of Russell (*loc. cit.*, *supra*) and others.

[24] ' Momentary ' is, of course, used in the sense of an interval of time extremely short in proportion to the total life span of human beings. The constitutional examination of an individual takes at least some hours. Theoretically, and sometimes actually, the man may be changing biologically to a significant degree even in that

time. Sigaud [*La forme humaine*. I. Sa significa-
tion, Paris and Lyon, 1914.] says (p. 5) : " Le fait
vivant évolue, c'est-à-dire décrit une trajectoire
composée d'une série de moments. L'observateur
ne saisit qu'un moment et ce moment varie
suivant les observations et suivant les observa-
teurs. En biologie, deux observations ne sont
jamais superposables ".

[25] Butler, S., *Life and Habit*, 1878 (Reprinted
1924), Chap. V, *passim*.

[26] Cuvier, G. L. C. F. D., *Le règne animal
distribué d'après son organisation, pour servir de
base à l'histoire naturelle des animaux et d'instruc-
tion à l'anatomie comparée*, Paris, 1817.

[27] This idea, in varying degrees of vagueness,
played a large rôle in the speculations of the
pre-Darwinian evolutionists. *Cf.* Pearl, R.,
" An eighteenth century French evolutionist ",
Human Biology, Vol. 2, pp. 559-566, 1930.

[28] For a more general biological discussion of
this point see Pearl, R., " On the distribution of
differences in vitality among individuals ", *Amer.
Nat.*, Vol. 61, pp. 113-131, 1927 ; and Pearl, R.,
The Rate of Living. New York, 1928.

[29] This appears to be as good a point as any to
list a few of the more important works in this
field, other than those already referred to elsewhere in these notes. The list is alphabetical by
authors. It makes no pretense to completeness.

Bauer, J. *Die konstitutionelle Disposition
zu inneren Krankheiten*, Zweite Aufl., Berlin,
1921.

Idem, *Vorlesungen über allgemeine Kon-
stitutions- und Vererbungslehre für Studierende
und Ärzte*, Zweite Aufl., Berlin, 1923.

Beneke, F. W., *Die anatomischen Grundlagen
der Constitutionsanomalien des Menschen*,
Marburg, 1878.

Idem, *Constitution und constitutionelles
Kranksein des Menschen*, Marburg, 1881.

Borel, Y., *Du diagnostic par le facies*, Thèse,
Fac. Med. No. 79. Montpellier, 1921. [The

illustrations in this thesis are charming—they amuse as well as inform.]

Brandt, W., *Grundzüge einer Konstitutionsanatomie*, Berlin, 1931. [This book has a very extensive bibliography of its subject, and is altogether a thoroughly sound and scholarly piece of work.]

Draper, G., *Human Constitution. A Consideration of its Relationship to Disease*, Philadelphia, 1924.

Idem, *Human Constitution, etc.*, Baltimore, 1928.

Idem, *Disease and the Man*, New York, 1930.

Hurst, A. F., *The Constitutional Factor* (Psyche Miniatures, Medical Series).

Krasusky, W. S., *Konstitutionstypen der Kinder*, Berlin, 1930.

Kretschmer, E., *Physique and Character. An Investigation of the Nature of Constitution and the Theory of Temperament.* Translated from the Second, Revised and Enlarged, Edition (International Library of Psychology), 1925.

Mac-Auliffe, L., *Les Tempéraments. Essai de Synthèse.* Paris, 1926.

Miller, E., *Types of Mind and Body* (Psyche Miniatures, Medical Series).

Naegeli, O., *Allgemeine Konstitutionslehre in naturwissenschaftlicher und medizinischer Betrachtung*, Berlin, 1927.

Pende, N. *Constitutional Inadequacies. An Introduction to the Study of Abnormal Constitution*, Translated by S. Naccarati, Philadelphia, 1928.

Thooris, A., *La Vie par le Stade*, Paris, 1924.

Wertheimer, F. I., and Florence E. Hesketh, *The Significance of the Physical Constitution in Mental Disease*, Baltimore, 1926.

[30] Wheeler, W. M., " The physiognomy of insects ", *Quart. Rev. Biol.*, Vol. 2, pp. 1-36, 1927.

This essay has been reprinted as one of the chapters in Prof. Wheeler's delightful *Foibles of Insects and Men*, New York, 1928.

[31] For a general discussion, with an extensive bibliography, of the biological consequences of differential relative growth of the parts of the animal body, a recent book by Julian S. Huxley (*Problems of Relative Growth*, New York, 1932) will be found interesting and useful. An important earlier treatise on the same subject by D'Arcy W. Thompson, [*Growth and Form*, Cambridge, 1917] is unfortunately out of print and difficult to come by.

[32] See Hoskins, R. G., *The Tides of Life. The Endocrine Glands in Bodily Adjustment*, New York, 1933. Also the following, written particularly for the practitioner, may be consulted : Cobb, I. G., *The Organs of Internal Secretion*, Fourth Edit., Baltimore, 1933.

[33] " The big Bogues ", *People*, Vol. 1, p. 45. This journal appears to have been a short-lived publication, but at least it served one useful purpose in putting on record this remarkable family.

[34] Tocher, J. F., " Anthropometric Observations on Samples of the Civil Population of Aberdeenshire, Banffshire, and Kincardineshire and A Study of the Chief Physical Characters of the Soldiers of Scottish Nationality and A Comparison with the Physical Characters of the Insane Population of Scotland " (*The William Ramsay Henderson Trust Reports*, Nos. II and III). Edinburgh, 1924.

[35] Galton, F., *Natural Inheritance, London*, 1889. This is the great pioneer treatise on the inheritance of the physical characters of man.

[36] Pearson, K., and Alice Lee, " On the laws of inheritance in man. I. Inheritance of physical characters ", *Biometrika*, Vol. 2, pp. 357-462, 1903.

[37] Davenport, C. B., " Body Build and its Inheritance ", *Carnegie Inst. of Washington*, Publ. No. 329.

[38] The great bulk of the work on the ideal or ' normal ' proportions of the human body has been done either by or for artists. In the nature

of the case there can, of course, be no absolute standard or criterion for the ' ideal ', or ' perfect ', or ' normal ' form of the human body except one that is either an expression (*a*) of folk taste, or (*b*) of a statistical concept which regards the mean or average of a group of human beings as the ' normal ' form. There is a considerable literature on the so-called ideal proportions of the body, which seems to have been unduly neglected by physical anthropologists. It may fairly be said to begin with Albrecht Dürer's treatise of 1528, '' Hierin sind begriffen vier Bücher von menschlicher Proportion durch Albrecht Dürer von Nürnberg erfunden und beschrieben zu nutz allen denen, so dieser Kunst lieb tragen ''. The first book on anthropometry, considered as a scientific subject and written for scientific ends and particularly those which would relate bodily habitus to health and disease, was Elscholtz's *Anthropometria* of 1654. A transcript of the title page of the first edition of this rare and important book is as follows : IOANNIS SIGISMVNDI / ELSHOLTII / ANTHROPOMETRIA / *Accessit* / DOCTRINA NAEVORVM. / AD / *Sereniss. S. R.I. Principem Electorem* / FRIDERICVM / GVILIELMVM / MARCHIONEM BRANDEBVRGICVM. / [Allegorical woodcut, surrounded by vignetted border, the whole 67 x 57.5 mm.] / [single rule, 119 mm.] / PATAVII, Typis Matthæi Cadorini / SVPERIORVM PERMISSV. / MDCLIV /. For some years past 1 have been working on a translation and annotated edition of this book, with the efficient aid of Miss Hermine Grimm. We hope that its completion and issue will not be much longer delayed. Coming down to more modern times one of the best treatises extant on the form and proportions of the human body is that of Gustav Fritsch, which appeared just at the end of the nineteenth century. The title page, which gives a good idea of the provenience and nature of the work, reads as follows : DIE / GESTALT DES MENSCHEN. / MIT BENUTZUNG DER WERKE / VON / E. HARLESS und C. SCHMIDT / FÜR KÜNSTLER UND ANTHROPOLOGEN DARGESTELLT /

VON / GUSTAV FRITSCH, / DR. MED., PRO-
FESSOR DER UNIVERSITÄT BERLIN, / GEHEIMER
MEDIZINALRATH./ [single rule, 18 mm.] / MIT
25 TAFELN UND 287 ABBILDUNGEN IM TEXT. /
[ornamental rule, 44 mm.] / STUTTGART, / PAUL
NEFF VERLAG. / [No date, but *Vorwort* dated
August 1899].

[39] I am very grateful to my former student,
Miss Barbara Jean Betz, M.S., and to my
colleague, Dr. John R. Miner, for their help in
the study of constitution and health upon which
the discussion here is based.

[40] This specification about reproductivity may
strike the reader as a curious one. The reason for
it is simply that I am engaged on an investigation of these same women from the viewpoint
of the relation between bodily habitus and
fertility, and have used the opportunity afforded
by so homogeneous a group to examine their
health records.

[41] Pearl, R., A. C. Sutton, W. T. Howard, Jr.,
and Margaret Rioch. " Studies on constitution.
I. Methods ", *Human Biology*, Vol. 1, pp.
10-56, 1929.

[42] Love, A. G., and L. J. Reed, " Biometric
Studies on U.S. Army Officers :
1. Longevity in relation to physical fitness ",
   *Proc. 21st Ann. Meet. Med. Sect. Amer.
   Life Conv., Washington, D.C.*, 1931.
2. " Somatological norms, correlations, and
   changes with age ", *Human Biol.*, Vol. 4,
   pp. 509-524, 1932.
3. " Somatological norms in disease ", *Human
   Biol.*, Vol. 5, pp. 61-93, 1933.
4. " Economic efficiency (length of service)
   in relation to physical fitness and other
   factors ", *Military Surg.*, Vol. 71, pp. 231-
   238, 1932.

[43] Imai, T. The influence of temperature on
variation and inheritance of bodily dimensions
in *Drosophila melanogaster, Arch. f. Entwicklungs-
mech.*, Bd. 128, pp. 634-660, 1933.

[44] Lishman, W. E., " The contribution of
cience to the future ", *Nature*, Vol. 130
p. 582, 1932.

PSYCHE

AN ANNUAL REVIEW
OF GENERAL AND APPLIED PSYCHOLOGY

Edited by C. K. OGDEN, M.A.
*(Editor of " The International Library of Psychology,
Philosophy, and Scientific Method")*

RECENT CONTRIBUTORS INCLUDE:

Dr. Alfred Adler
Prof. Charles Baudouin
J. D. Bernal
Dr. William Brown
Prof. S. Buchanan
Prof. E. Bugnion
Dr. Trigant Burrow
Prof. Cyril Burt
Dr. F. G. Crookshank
E. J. Dingwall
Prof. Auguste Forel
Prof. M. Ginsberg
Dr. R. G. Gordon
Dr. H. Hartridge
Prof. Lancelot Hogben
Prof. Pierre Janet
Prof. Otto Jespersen
Dr. Ernest Jones
Prof. K. Koffka
Prof. Laignel-Lavastine

Miss L. W. Lockhart
William McDougall, F.R.S.
Prof. Bronislaw Malinowski
Dr. E. Miller
Dr. T. W. Mitchell
Dr. C. S. Myers, F.R.S.
Dr. Oscar Oeser
Prof. F. Paulhan
Prof. T. H. Pear
Prof. H. Piéron
Dr. I. A. Richards
Bertrand Russell, F.R.S.
Prof. Sante De Sanctis
Prof. E. Sapir
Prof. G. Elliot Smith, F.R.S.
Vilhjalmur Stefansson
Baron von Uexküll
Dr. John B. Watson
Prof. W. M. Wheeler
Dr. William A. White

Price 10/-

A few bound sets of PSYCHE, Vols. I—XII, 1920—1932, are
still available, price £15 the set

PSYCHE

10, KING'S PARADE, CAMBRIDGE, ENGLAND

BASIC ENGLISH

Basic English
A general account, with Word-list and Rules.

The Basic Words
A full account of the 850, with all special uses.

The A B C of Basic English
A simple account, step by step, for learners and teachers.

The Basic Dictionary
Putting into Basic the 7,500 words most used in Normal English

The Basic Vocabulary
A history and discussion of the question; with details of the number of words used for different purposes.

Debabelization
The argument for Basic as the international language of the future; with over 100 pages of current opinion on the position of English.

Brighter Basic .
For young persons of taste and feeling. This is not a book for teachers, but it may be of value to those who are tired and sad.

Basic for Business
A complete system for international trade, with examples of business letters for all purposes.

Basic English Applied : Science
Taking the learner to a stage where international words are ready to hand. Chemistry, Physics, and Biology are here covered

Basic for Economics
Covering economic theory; with examples from representative writers.

EXAMPLES

Basic by Examples. Every Basic word with its different uses.
The Basic Traveller. Simple examples for all purposes.
The Gold Insect. Poe's "Gold Bug" put into Basic English.
Julius Caesar. From North's Plutarch (with "Brutus").
Robinson Crusoe. His story in Basic.
Japanese Stories. From Lafcadio Hearn.
That Night. Tumura's "Sono Yo" in Basic.
The Organization of Peace. By Maxwell Garnett.
International Talks. By Wickham Steed; with Basic parallel.
Lamb's Stories from Shakespeare. A Basic selection.
Stories from the Bible. A selection from the coming Basic Bible.
The Chemical History of a Candle. Faraday in Basic.
Black Beauty. Anna Sewell's story. For school use.
Carl and Anna. Leonhard Frank's story. Not for school use.

THE ORTHOLOGICAL INSTITUTE

10, KING'S PARADE, CAMBRIDGE, ENGLAND
LONDON: KEGAN PAUL, 68, CARTER LANE, E.C